Vegan cook
People

Vegan High protein meals with easy and specific steps. Lose weight fast and Heal your body with easy recipes

Written By

JANE BRACE

Table of Contents

CHOCOLATE-COVERED PECAN PIE COOKIES 43

APRICOT COOKIES 45

CINNAMON AMARETTI 46

CITRUS-KISSED MACAROONS 48

PEANUT BUTTER CHOCOLATE CHIA PUDDING 49

CHOCO-CADO PUDDING 50

RAW CHOCOLATE 55

COCONUTTY CANDY 56

ALMOND BON BONS 57

RAISINETTE BONBONS 59

NOURISHING BROWNIE BITES 60

CHOCOLATE NANAIMO BARS 62

CHOCOLATE GRANOLA 67

SWEET, SALTY, AND SOFT GRANOLA BARS 68

POWERHOUSE BARS 70

CHERRY PIE BARS 72

CHERRY CHOCOLATE ALMOND SNACK BARS 73

PEANUT BUTTER BANANA ICE CREAM 77

FRESH FRUITSICLES 78

FRUIT SALSA AND CINNAMON CRISPS 79

TRUFFLES AND FUDGE

SALTED ESPRESSO TRUFFLES

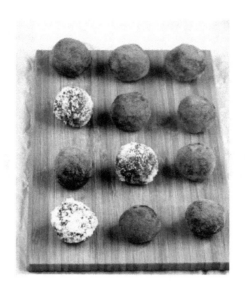

YIELD: 36 TRUFFLES

The first chocolate truffle is speculated to have originated in France, but today, there are countless varieties from countless countries, making it one of the most popular chocolates in the world. The secret to a perfect truffle is the ratio: 2 parts chocolate to 1 part cream.

1 cup couverture chocolate or non dairy chocolate chips

½ cup canned full-fat coconut milk

⅛ teaspoon sea salt

1 teaspoon vanilla extract

½ teaspoon espresso powder

½ cup cocoa powder or almond meal, for dusting

- Over a double boiler, melt the couverture until completely smooth. Remove bowl from heat and place on a heat-safe surface.

- In a small saucepan, warm the coconut milk, salt, vanilla extract, and espresso powder just until it begins to simmer and is obviously hot to the touch, but do not let it come to a boil.

- Using a whisk, gently stir the warmed coconut milk mixture into the center of the melted couverture and blend gently and carefully in a circular fashion until completely mixed. Transfer mixture to a plastic bowl and cover with plastic wrap.

- Chill in refrigerator for about 1 to 2 hours, until firm.

- Using a small scoop or rounded spoon, and chocolate-dusted hands, roll the chocolate into 1-inch balls. Immediately roll the truffles into the cocoa powder. Chill before serving and store in airtight container in the refrigerator for up to 2 weeks.

STRAWBERRY PISTACHIO TRUFFLES

YIELD: 25 TRUFFLES

What a fantastic flavor combination strawberry and pistachio make along with chocolate. Feel free to use homemade Strawberry Preserves or store-bought—both will taste equally as divine.

2 cups non dairy semi-sweet chocolate chips

¼ cup + 2 tablespoons full-fat coconut milk

1 teaspoon vanilla extract

¼ cup strawberry preserves

1 cup pistachios, chopped finely

* In a saucepan over medium-low heat, combine all of the ingredients except for the pistachios.

* Stir constantly until the chocolate is fully melted and the mixture is very well combined.

* Transfer to a bowl and chill just until it's easy to work into a ball, for about 2 hours. A quick trip to the freezer will help them out as well.

* Using a 1-inch ice cream scoop, form chocolate into balls and then roll into the chopped pistachios. Place onto a parchment-covered plate or tray and chill overnight in refrigerator or until firm. Store in airtight container in refrigerator for up to 1 month.

CHERRY CORDIALS

YIELD: 15 TO 20 CANDIES

These candies are simple to make but do require tempered couverture and chocolate molds to make them work, as untempered chocolate is too soft and no molds will cause messy cordials. For a quick refresher on how to temper chocolate, refer to <u>tempering</u>.

15 to 20 maraschino cherries, stems removed (see note)

¼ cup brandy

1 cup couverture, tempered

⅓ cup + 1 tablespoon confectioners sugar

3 teaspoons cherry juice (from cherry jar)

¼ teaspoon vanilla or almond extract

A chocolate mold

- Drain the liquid from the maraschino cherries, set it aside, and place the cherries on a paper towel. Transfer the cherries into a small bowl containing the brandy and allow to soak for 1 hour. Remove from brandy and place onto a dry paper towel. Let the cherries rest until they are fairly dry to the touch, for about 1 hour.

- Brush the tempered chocolate onto the insides of the chocolate mold to coat the sides evenly. Let chocolate completely harden. Place one cherry into each cavity.

- Mix together the confectioner's sugar, cherry juice, and vanilla extract and pour a small amount (just to fill) on top of the cherries. Top with tempered chocolate and let rest until chocolate has completely hardened. Store in airtight container for up to 1 week.

ALLERGY NOTE

Use vanilla extract instead of almond for a nut-free candy.

You can also omit the fondant filling and just dip the brandy soaked cherries straight into the tempered couverture. This works especially well if you leave the stems on the cherries. Just dip and place onto waxed paper to harden.

BUCKEYES

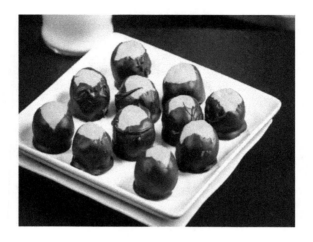

YIELD: 30 BUCKEYES

You can use chocolate chips with these or couverture. Born and raised in Ohio, I tend to think the chocolate chip method is more authentic, but, admittedly, the couverture is definitely more glamorous and adds a nice shell to the outer layer. Be sure when dipping to leave a little bit of peanut butter exposed (about ½ inch in diameter) so that the candies resemble actual buckeyes!

1½ cups smooth peanut butter

1 cup non dairy margarine, softened to room temperature

2 teaspoons vanilla extract

¼ teaspoon salt

5¾ to 6 cups confectioners sugar

3 cups non dairy chocolate chips or couverture

- Line a 9 × 13-inch cookie sheet with waxed paper.

- Mix together peanut butter and margarine until super smooth.

- Stir in vanilla extract and salt.

- Using electric mixer, slowly incorporate the confectioner's sugar until little crumbles form. The mixture should go from very creamy to looking like pulverized very crumbly dry cookie dough.

- Take a pinch or two of the powder/dough and, using your hands, work to form into 1-inch balls. If they appear uneven, keep working them in your hands until smooth and spherical.

- Place each onto a cookie sheet and insert a toothpick into the center. Gently pat around the toothpick to kind of "seal" it into the peanut butter ball.

- Chill in freezer for about 40 minutes, or until very firm. This prevents the toothpicks from sliding out while dipping.

- Using a double boiler, melt your chocolate until smooth or follow the directions for tempering. Remove the peanut butter balls from the freezer and carefully swirl the ball into the chocolate, taking care not to let the toothpick slide out. Place onto wax paper and repeat until all are covered. Let stand at room temperature until chocolate has firmed up. Remove toothpicks and seal over the tiny hole in the middle using the back of a spoon or clean fingertips. Store in airtight container for up to 1 month.

17

DARK AND DREAMY FUDGE

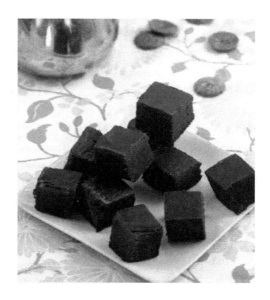

YIELD: 64 PIECES

Super rich and extra dreamy, this fudge is best enjoyed in small pieces so that you can savor the intense flavor. If you like some crunch in your fudge, simply add 1 cup of toasted walnut pieces into the fudge before spreading into a prepared pan, or sprinkle on top.

½ cup sugar

1 teaspoon vanilla extract

2 tablespoons non dairy milk

2 tablespoons non dairy margarine

10 ounces Ricemellow (vegan marshmallow) Cream

3 cups non dairy chocolate chips

- Prepare an 8 × 8-inch pan by lightly greasing with non dairy margarine.

- In a 2-quart saucepan, combine the sugar, vanilla extract, nondairy milk, and margarine and bring to a boil over medium heat. Cook for 1 minute, stirring often. Stir in the Ricemellow Cream and heat just until warm and all of it has evenly combined with the sugar mixture, for about 4 minutes.

- Quickly stir in the chocolate chips until they have completely melted and pour the mixture into the prepared pan. Let cool completely and then chill in the refrigerator for at least 2 hours before cutting. Store in an airtight container in the refrigerator for up to 1 month.

PEANUT BUTTER FUDGE

YIELD: 20 PIECES

This is a perfect choice for when you're craving candy, but don't have a candy thermometer handy. Working quickly is an important part of making this fudge, so be sure to have all your ingredients and equipment ready before you begin.

½ cup non dairy margarine

2 cups brown sugar

½ cup non dairy milk

1 cup creamy peanut butter

1½ teaspoons vanilla extract

3 cups confectioners sugar

1½ cups non dairy chocolate chips

- Lightly grease a standard-size loaf pan or small square cake pan.

- In a 2-quart saucepan, over medium heat, warm the margarine until melted. Add the brown sugar and nondairy milk and cook over medium heat until mixture comes to a hard boil (for about 2 to 3 minutes).

- Once it comes to a hard boil, set your timer for exactly 2 minutes. Continue to cook over medium heat, stirring the entire time it is cooking, washing down sugar crystals as needed.

- After 2 minutes, remove from the heat and quickly stir in your peanut butter and vanilla extract, and promptly add the confectioner's sugar, mixing briefly just until all the sugar has been incorporated.

- Spread the thick candy into prepared pan and wait for it to set up slightly.

- Once the fudge has cooled slightly, melt chocolate chips over a double boiler and drizzle all over the fudge. Let chocolate reharden and then serve! Store in airtight container for up to 2 weeks.

FRUIT-BASED CANDIES

SUGAR PLUMS

YIELD: 24 SUGAR PLUMS

These little gems have become well known from their very important cameo in the classic Christmas tale, and, even though they may conjure up images of sugar-covered plums in your mind, they actually have never contained any plums at all. "Plum" used to be a popular way to describe any dried fruit, but sugar plums usually contained a mixture of dates, apricots, or figs to achieve their sweetness.

1 cup raw almonds

1 teaspoon lemon or orange zest

½ cup chopped dried figs

½ cup chopped dried dates

½ teaspoon cinnamon

¼ teaspoon nutmeg

Dash ground cloves

2 tablespoons agave

½ cup confectioners sugar for dusting

- Preheat oven to 400°F and spread the almonds in an even layer on a cookie sheet. Bake for 7 minutes, or until fragrant.

- Place almonds, zest, figs, dates, cinnamon, nutmeg, and cloves into a food processor and pulse until crumbly. Add in the agave, 1 tablespoon at a time, and pulse again, until the mixture comes together easily. Pinch into 1-inch balls and roll in the confectioner's sugar. Store in airtight container for up to 1 week.

ALLERGY NOTE

For a nut-free variation, try these with toasted sunflower seeds, hemp seeds, or even flaked coconut in place of the almonds.

CANDIED ORANGE PEELS

YIELD: 3 CUPS

Candied orange peels are so nice to have for decorative purposes or to add a little zing to a dessert, like in my Florentines. This recipe also works nicely with lemon or lime peels, which add a nice color variation to the mix.

4 navel oranges

1½ cups sugar

¾ cup water

Dash salt

- Remove the peels from the oranges by slicing through the peel and quartering it, without puncturing the fruit. Gently cut off the top and bottom of the orange and then carefully peel the orange peel, leaving behind the pith and fruit. Reserve pith and fruit for another use (these make fantastic juicing oranges).

- Lay one section of peel flat onto a cutting area, light-side-up. Slice the peel into thin, even strips, about ¼ inch wide.

- Place the peels into a medium saucepan and cover with 1 inch of water and salt very lightly. Boil for 20 minutes, and then drain. Briefly place onto clean kitchen towel to dry.

- Drain the saucepan and then wipe dry. Place the drained peels, sugar, water, and salt into the pot and cook over medium heat. Cook until the mixture reaches 235°F on a candy thermometer (or Soft Ball Stage if using the Cold

26

Water Method). Spread in an even layer onto a waxed paper–covered cookie sheet or silicone mat. Let harden for 2 hours, and for up to 12 hours before transferring to airtight container. Store for up to 1 month.

SOUR FRUIT JELLIES

YIELD: 30 CANDIES

These jelly candies are a touch softer than traditional gumdrops. They actually taste more like fruit snacks made for children's lunches.

¾ cup white grape juice

⅓ cup fruit pectin

½ teaspoon baking soda

1 cup sugar

1 cup agave

1 to 2 drops food coloring, any color

¼ teaspoon citric acid

⅓ cup turbinado sugar

- Line an 8 × 8-inch pan snugly with aluminum foil and spray generously with nonstick spray or grease with margarine.

- In a small saucepan, over medium heat, warm the grape juice, pectin, and baking soda just until boiling. Once boiling, reduce heat to lowest setting, stirring occasionally.

- In a 2-quart saucepan, whisk together the sugar and agave and cook over medium heat, until it reaches 265°F on a candy thermometer (or Hard Ball Stage if using the Cold Water Method). Be sure to stir occasionally while this mixture is cooking, and, once the sugar dissolves, brush down the sides with a wet pastry brush to remove any crystals.

- After the sugar mixture has reached 265°F, stir in the grape juice mixture along with the desired shade of food coloring. You can easily separate these into various colors by pouring the mixture into separate bowls and coloring each a different color. Pour into the prepared pan (or pans if making multiple colors) and chill in refrigerator overnight. Remove from refrigerator and cut into shapes using a very small cookie cutters. Mix the citric acid and turbinado sugar in a small bowl and dip the cut candies to coat. Store in refrigerator in airtight container for up to 1 month.

Citric acid, which adds the sour flavor, can be located in most supermarkets next to canning goods. Of course, you could always leave the citric acid out and keep them sugary sweet instead.

NATURE'S CANDY: REFINED SUGAR–FREE TREATS

This chapter captures the essence of sweet, without the need for any refined sweeteners. Instead, I've come up with a slew of recipes that utilize fruits and other refined sugar–free sweeteners such as maple syrup, agave, and stevia, and many of them use whole fruit, adding a few key nutrients in there for good measure. These desserts are especially good for little ones who may be craving something extra sweet, but don't need all the extra sugar. For recipes calling for Sweetened Whipped Coconut Cream, refer to the recipe and use the stevia variation.

COOKIES AND OTHER FAMILIAR FAVORITES

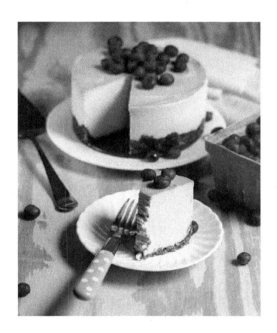

PUMPKIN MUFFINS

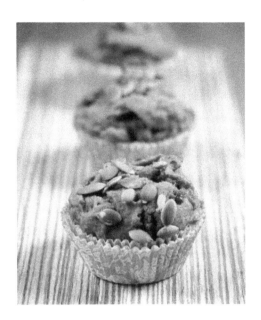

YIELD: 12 MUFFINS

These tender morsels are studded with raw pumpkin seeds, called pepitas, to add a delightful color and texture to the muffins.

1¼ cups brown rice flour

½ cup potato starch

¼ cup tapioca flour

1 teaspoon xanthan gum

¼ teaspoon baking soda

1 teaspoon baking powder

1 teaspoon salt

1 teaspoon cinnamon

1 cup coconut palm sugar

¼ cup olive or coconut oil

1 cup pumpkin puree

⅓ cup + 2 tablespoons non dairy milk

2 tablespoons apple cider vinegar

½ cup pepitas

- Preheat oven to 400°F and line a muffin pan with twelve liners, lightly spritz with nonstick spray, or simply grease a standard-size muffin pan.

- In a large bowl, whisk together the brown rice flour, potato starch, tapioca flour, xanthan gum, baking soda, baking powder, salt, cinnamon, and coconut palm sugar. Stir in the oil, pumpkin puree, nondairy milk, and apple cider vinegar and mix until smooth. Fold in the pepitas. Divide batter evenly among the twelve cups and bake for about 20 minutes, or until a knife inserted into the center comes out clean. Store in airtight container for up to 3 days.

BANANA NUT MUFFINS

YIELD: 12 MUFFINS

These muffins are just too darn delicious with the warm flavor of banana and walnuts. Be sure to grease the muffin liners on these, or use silicone muffin cups; since these muffins contain very little oil, they may have a tendency to stick.

¾ cup brown rice flour

½ cup potato starch

¼ cup tapioca flour

1 teaspoon xanthan gum

1½ teaspoons baking powder

¼ teaspoon baking soda

¼ teaspoon salt

1 teaspoon vanilla extract

3 mashed bananas, about 1⅓ cups

⅓ cup + 1 tablespoon maple syrup

2 tablespoons olive oil

2 tablespoons vinegar

½ cup chopped walnuts

- Preheat oven to 350°F. Using margarine or coconut oil, grease twelve standard-size muffin cups, or spritz twelve liners with nonstick spray.

- In a medium bowl, whisk together the brown rice flour, potato starch, tapioca flour, xanthan gum, baking powder, baking soda, and salt. Make a well in the center and stir in the vanilla extract, bananas, maple syrup, olive oil, and vinegar. Stir the mixture until very well combined and then fold in the walnuts.

- Divide the batter evenly among the muffin cups and bake for 30 minutes, until golden brown on edges. Let cool completely before serving. Store in airtight container for up to 3 days.

These muffins take exceptionally well to a few cacao nibs added to the batter before baking.

LEMON POPPYSEED SCONES

YIELD: 12 SCONES

Scones have always intrigued me with their not quite biscuity, not quite cakey demeanor. I don't exactly want to eat them for breakfast but they always seem perfect for a midday snacking.

⅓ cup almond flour

⅓ cup corn flour

1 cup millet flour

½ cup brown rice flour

½ cup tapioca flour

1 teaspoon xanthan gum

2 teaspoons baking powder

1 teaspoon baking soda

½ teaspoon salt

½ cup nonhydrogenated vegetable shortening

½ cup maple syrup

1 tablespoon flaxseed meal

2 tablespoons water

½ cup lemon juice

2 tablespoons poppyseed

1 tablespoon lemon zest

- Preheat oven to 375°F. Mix the almond flour, corn flour, millet flour, brown rice flour, and tapioca flour together in large mixing bowl. Stir in xanthan gum, baking powder, baking soda, and salt.

- Cut in the shortening using your hands, until it forms equal-size crumbles. Add in maple syrup. In a small bowl, combine the flaxseed meal and water and let rest until thickened, for about 5 minutes.

- Using a fork, combine the prepared flaxseed meal with the rest of the ingredients until the mixture becomes evenly crumbly.

- Still using a fork, mix in the lemon juice, poppyseed, and lemon zest. Once dough becomes well mixed, turn out onto a lightly floured surface (millet flour is recommended) and gently fold over about three times. Roll about ¾ inch thick and cut into squares using a sharp knife. You can also use a biscuit cutter to make circles. Place onto ungreased cookie sheet.

- Bake for about 13 minutes or until golden brown on top. Store in airtight container for up to 1 week.

GINGERBREAD SQUARES

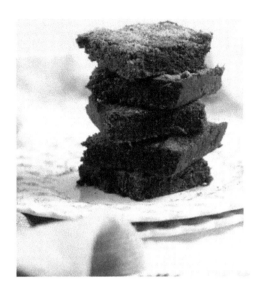

YIELD: 8 SERVINGS

Sweetened by banana, blackstrap molasses, and agave, this healthy gingerbread tastes just as rich and spicy as the traditional version.

1 ripe banana, mashed

2 tablespoons blackstrap (or regular) molasses

1 teaspoon freshly grated ginger

1 teaspoon cinnamon

¼ teaspoon cloves

¼ teaspoon salt

2 tablespoons agave or maple syrup

2 tablespoons ground chia seed

1 cup almond meal

⅓ cup teff flour

- In a large bowl, stir together the banana, molasses, ginger, cinnamon, cloves, salt, and agave until smooth. Fold in the chia seed, almond meal, and teff flour. Lightly grease a 4 × 8-inch loaf pan and spread the mixture into the pan. Bake for 30 minutes. Let cool completely and then slice into squares. Store in an airtight container for up to 1 week.

SWEET CORNCAKE COOKIES

YIELD: 12 COOKIES

Corn adds a sweet touch as well as a nice color to these cookies, which can be made with maple syrup or agave. Masa harina can be found in Mexican groceries or in most grocery stores along with the Mexican ingredients.

2 tablespoons flaxseed meal

4 tablespoons water

¾ cup fine yellow cornmeal

½ cup maple syrup or agave

½ teaspoon salt

½ cup masa harina

¼ cup white rice flour

¼ cup tapioca flour

1 tablespoon olive oil

- Preheat oven to 350°F. Line a cookie sheet with parchment or a silicone mat. In a small bowl, mix the flaxseed meal with water and allow to rest until gelled, for about 5 minutes. Mix together all the ingredients in a medium bowl in the order listed, scraping sides of bowl well while mixing.

- Drop by the tablespoonful onto the prepared cookie sheet and flatten slightly with the back of a fork. Bake for 12 to 15 minutes.

- Let cool completely before serving. Store in airtight container in refrigerator for up to 1 week.

CHOCOLATE-COVERED PECAN PIE COOKIES

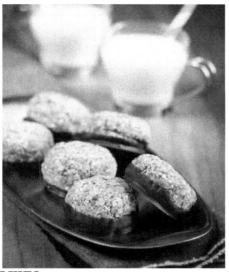

YIELD: 20 COOKIES

With chia seed and nuts, these delicious cookies taste sinful but are made from surprisingly wholesome ingredients. For a slightly more convenient version (and almost refined sugar–free), use non dairy chocolate chips for dipping the bottoms of the cookies instead of Raw Chocolate.

2 teaspoons ground chia seed

2 tablespoons water

1½ cups raw pecans

1 cup raw cashews

¼ cup coconut flour

½ teaspoon salt 6 dates

¾ cup <u>Raw Chocolate</u>, melted

- Preheat oven to 325°F. In a small bowl, mix together the chia seed and water and let rest until gelled, for about 5 minutes.

- Place the pecans, cashews, coconut flour, and salt into a food processor and blend until crumbly, for about 1 minute. Do not overmix! Once crumbly, add the dates, two at a time, until the mixture clumps together easily. Process just until dates are well mixed. Shape into disks 1½ inches wide by ½ inch thick and place onto an ungreased cookie sheet. Bake for 15 minutes.

- Let cool and then dip bottoms of cookies into the Raw Chocolate, placing back onto a silicone mat or wax paper–covered baking sheet. Chill for about 20 minutes in refrigerator until the chocolate has set. Store in airtight container for up to 1 week.

APRICOT COOKIES

YIELD: 18 COOKIES

These golden, chewy, slightly sweet cookies are just as easy to prepare as they are to eat! Packed with vitamins A and C from the apricots and protein and iron from the walnuts and coconut, these cookies are like snack-size energy bars.

3 cups dried apricots

1 cup walnut pieces

2 cups unsweetened shredded coconut, plus about ⅓ cup for rolling

¼ cup agave

- Combine all ingredients (set aside ⅓ cup coconut) in a food processor and process until very well chopped.

- Using clean hands, roll the mixture into walnut-size balls and then into the extra coconut. Flatten into cookie rounds using the bottom of a glass or measuring cup, and then gently shape with hands to create even patties.

- Store in airtight container for up to 1 week.

CINNAMON AMARETTI

YIELD: 36 COOKIES

Amaretti are classic small Italian cookies that are crisp on the outside and a bit chewier in the center—and one of my favorite cookies of all. You won't miss the refined sugar in this version. For best texture, shape the cookies into small mounds, about 1 inch across, for perfect chewy-center-to-crispy-outside ratio.

3 tablespoons flaxseed meal

6 tablespoons water

3 cups almond meal

1½ teaspoons cinnamon

1¼ cups coconut palm sugar

¾ teaspoon salt

Sliced almonds, for garnish

- Preheat oven to 300°F. Line a large baking sheet with parchment paper.

- In a small bowl, combine the flaxseed meal with the water and let rest for 5 minutes, until gelled. Transfer to a large bowl and stir in the almond meal, cinnamon, palm sugar, and salt. Keep stirring until the mixture comes together into a stiff dough; it may not appear to be coming together, but keep stirring! This is also done effortlessly using an electric mixer.

- When the dough stiffens, pinch off 1-inch sections and form into rounds.

Place onto the cookie sheet about 1 inch apart and top with a sliced almond. Bake for 30 minutes. Let cool completely. Store in airtight container for up to 1 week.

CITRUS-KISSED MACAROONS

YIELD: 18 COOKIES

Lightly touched with lemon, these macaroons have only a handful of ingredients and don't need to be baked. They make a great snack post- workout or when the midday munchies arise.

12 Medjool dates, pitted

1 tablespoon lemon juice

2 tablespoons water

4 cups unsweetened shredded coconut, divided

- Combine the Medjool dates, lemon juice, and water in a food processor and blend until very smooth, scraping down the sides as necessary. Add 1 cup shredded coconut and pulse until very well combined.

- Transfer to a large bowl and by hand incorporate the additional 3 cups coconut until evenly mixed. Form the mixture into cookies and place onto cookie sheet. Refrigerate briefly to set.

- Store in an airtight container for up to 2 weeks.

PEANUT BUTTER CHOCOLATE CHIA PUDDING

YIELD: 2 SERVINGS

This dessert is as easy as pie (or pudding) to make, and it's healthy, filling, and delicious, too. Adjust sugar levels to your taste preferences, erring on the low side of things.

3 tablespoons whole chia seed, white or black

½ cup water

2 tablespoons non dairy milk (I recommend almond or coconut)

1 tablespoon cocoa powder

3 tablespoons creamy peanut butter

1½ tablespoons coconut date syrup or maple syrup

* Place all ingredients into a small to medium bowl and stir vigorously with a fork until smooth. Transfer into desired serving dishes and chill in refrigerator until gelled, for about 30 minutes. Best if served cold with a dollop of whipped coconut cream. Keeps for up to 1 day if stored in airtight container in the refrigerator.

CHOCO-CADO PUDDING

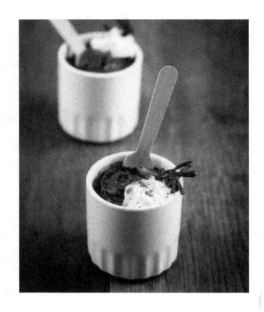

YIELD: 4 SERVINGS

Here's another surprise ingredient from the plant world: avocado is the superstar here, making a creamy base for this insanely rich chocolate pudding.

2 ripe avocados, pitted and peeled

¼ cup <u>Date Syrup</u> or agave

3 tablespoons coconut sugar

¼ cup cocoa powder

½ teaspoon espresso powder

¼ teaspoon salt

- Blend all ingredients together into a food processor until fluffy. Serve with whipped coconut cream! Store in airtight container in refrigerator for up to 3 days.

CLASSIC-STYLE
SWEETS

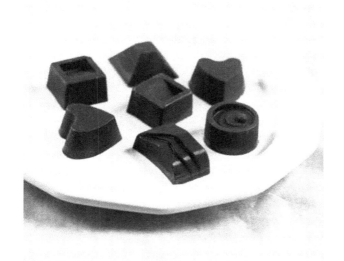

RAW CHOCOLATE

YIELD: 12 CANDIES

This chocolate can be molded using a chocolate mold or drizzled onto desserts for a chocolaty coating. Feel free to control the sweetness to your liking without affecting the final texture too much.

½ cup melted cacao butter

⅓ cup + 2 tablespoons cocoa powder

⅓ cup agave or maple syrup Pinch salt

* Whisk together all of the ingredients into a medium bowl. Pour the mixture into molds and rap on a solid flat surface to remove any air bubbles. Chill in the refrigerator until solid. To use as a coating, simply melt all ingredients back down and whisk well to combine. Store in airtight container in refrigerator for up to 1 week.

COCONUTTY CANDY

YIELD: 24 PIECES

This subtly sweet treat is nuts over coconut, in that it is made entirely out of coconut, save the vanilla extract and salt. To cut easily, let the solid candy thaw at room temperature for about 20 minutes before slicing and then returning to the refrigerator.

12 ounces (about 2½ cups) unsweetened shredded coconut

½ cup softened coconut oil, unrefined

1 teaspoon vanilla extract

½ cup coconut palm sugar

⅛ teaspoon salt

- In a blender or food processor, blend the coconut until smooth like peanut butter. This could take anywhere from 3 to 10 minutes, depending on your appliance, the dryness of the coconut, and temperature, among other factors. Just blend until smooth, and, if it never gets smooth, add a teaspoon or two of coconut oil to move things along.

- Once the shredded coconut has blended, add the remaining ingredients and blend until smooth. Pour into an 8 × 8-inch square dish, cover loosely with plastic wrap, and freeze for 30 minutes. Cut into small squares, and transfer to the refrigerator to store for up to 2 weeks.

ALMOND BON BONS

These are such a fun treat to snack on when a chocolate craving hits. Make a batch and store in the freezer—you can just grab one whenever you're in need of a little mood boost!

FILLING

1 cup almond meal

2 tablespoons coconut oil, softened

2 tablespoons agave, brown rice, or maple syrup

3 tablespoons melted cacao butter

⅛ teaspoon salt

COATING

1 recipe Raw Chocolate, melted

- In a medium bowl, combine all the filling ingredients and let rest for about 10 minutes. Shape into balls or place into silicone chocolate molds and then chill for about 30 minutes in the refrigerator, or for 10 minutes in the freezer, until solid.

- Once the filling is cold, dip the balls into the chocolate coating until completely covered, and then place coated truffles onto a silicone mat or parchment-covered surface to harden. Dip once more in the chocolate coating and then allow the chocolate to harden completely in the refrigerator, for about 1 hour. Store in airtight container in refrigerator for up to 1 month, or in freezer bags, tightly sealed, for up to 3 months.

RAISINETTE BONBONS

YIELD: ABOUT 20 BONBONS

These taste so much like the popular candies, it certainly won't seem like you're eating something so good for you!

1½ cups raisins

1 cup walnuts

¼ cup cocoa powder

- In a food processor, combine all the ingredients and blend until finely ground and clumped together, for about 1 minute. Roll into bite-size balls and place in refrigerator to chill for about 30 minutes prior to enjoying. Store in airtight container in refrigerator for up to 2 weeks.

NOURISHING BROWNIE BITES

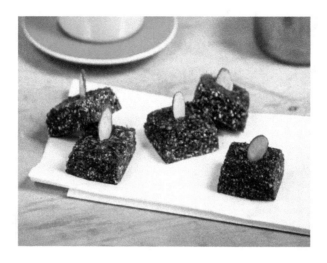

YIELD: 12 SERVINGS

In terms of brownies, this version is much healthier than your typical chocolaty square, but they sure don't miss a beat taste-wise. You won't feel bad about going back for seconds with these, as they are packed full of healthy stuff like dates, which contain fiber; cashews, which are high in magnesium; and cocoa, which is high in iron.

10 Medjool dates, chilled in fridge

2 cups whole cashews, unroasted

2 tablespoons cocoa powder

½ teaspoon salt

2 teaspoons vanilla extract

- Remove the pits from the dates and place into a food processor along with the cashews, cocoa powder, and salt. Pulse several times to combine and then blend until very crumbly, for about 2 minutes. Once the mixture is evenly crumbly, with the consistency of a coarse sugar, drizzle in the vanilla extract and continue to blend until the mixture becomes clumpy.

- Depending on the size and moisture content of your dates, you may need to add a touch more liquid, such as water or more vanilla extract, or process for a shorter amount of time to get the right consistency. In the end, the dough should easily stick together when balled. If it is too dry, add a bit more liquid (½ teaspoon or so) and if it is too wet, add in a tablespoon more cocoa powder to dry it out.

- Place the dough into the center of a parchment paper and cover with another sheet. Roll out gently to flatten into an even shape and then cut into squares. Chill in refrigerator for at least 20 minutes before serving. Store in airtight container in refrigerator for up to 2 weeks.

CHOCOLATE NANAIMO BARS

YIELD: 16 SERVINGS

Nanaimo bars, named after the city in British Columbia, are a popular no- bake dessert that are typically made with a LOT of butter and sugar. If you're not concerned about them being totally sugar-free, you can also use your favorite non dairy chocolate chips/buttons in place of the raw chocolate.

CRUST

1 cup whole raw almonds

10 dates

1 tablespoon cocoa powder

FILLING

2 cups cashews, soaked 2 hours

1½ teaspoons vanilla extract

⅔ cup coconut oil, melted

1 teaspoon stevia powder

3 Medjool dates or ¼ cup Date Syrup

2 tablespoons coconut cream (from the top of a chilled can of coconut milk)

TOPPING

1¼ cups Raw Chocolate, melted

* To make the crust, in a food processor, pulse together the almonds, five of

the dates, and the cocoa powder until crumbly. Add in the remaining five dates and pulse again until evenly chopped. Press the mixture firmly into an 8 × 8-inch baking pan.

- Make the filling in a food processor by combining the cashews, vanilla, coconut oil, stevia, dates, and coconut cream until very smooth, for about 5 minutes, scraping down sides as needed. Spread the filling evenly on top of the crust by using a flat silicone spatula. Freeze for 1 hour and then cut into squares.

- Top with melted chocolate and then return to freezer. Chill in freezer overnight, or for at least 6 hours. Store in refrigerator in airtight container for up to 2 weeks.

SNACK BARS AND GRANOLA

CHOCOLATE GRANOLA

YIELD: 3 CUPS

This versatile granola is perfect for all sorts of treats: Use for parfaits or to top your favorite non dairy yogurt or ice cream. Great in a bowl as breakfast cereal at home, or as a chocolaty addition to your trail mix when you're on the go.

2 cups certified gluten-free oats

⅓ cup almond meal

3 tablespoons whole chia seed

¼ teaspoon salt

⅓ cup cocoa powder

1 tablespoon coconut oil

1 teaspoon vanilla extract

⅓ cup agave or maple syrup

* Preheat oven to 300°F. In a medium bowl, whisk together the oats, almond meal, chia seed, salt, and cocoa powder. In a smaller bowl, whisk together the coconut oil, vanilla extract, and maple syrup until very smooth. Using clean hands, or a large fork, combine all ingredients until well mixed. Spread onto a parchment-lined jelly roll pan and bake for 40 minutes. Break into bite-size pieces and let cool completely. Store in airtight container for up to 3 weeks.

SWEET, SALTY, AND SOFT GRANOLA BARS

YIELD: 12 BARS

With its salty, sweet flavor and soft, chewy texture, this snack can satisfy multiple cravings at once! Store in an airtight container in the refrigerator for best texture.

2½ cups certified gluten-free oats

½ cup almond meal

1 teaspoon salt

2 tablespoons maple syrup

⅓ cup agave

¼ cup + 2 tablespoons softened coconut oil

¼ cup date sugar or coconut palm sugar

1 teaspoon vanilla extract

½ cup sliced almonds

1 tablespoon ground chia seed

3 tablespoons water

- Preheat oven to 350°F. Lightly grease an 8 × 8-inch pan.

- Spread the oats in an even layer onto a large baking sheet and lightly toast for 7 minutes. Remove oats from the oven and place them in a large mixing bowl. Using your hands, crumble in the almond meal, salt, maple syrup, agave, coconut oil, date sugar, vanilla extract, and sliced almonds.

- Mix the chia seed and water and let rest for 5 minutes, until gelled. Mix in with the rest of the ingredients and then using hands lightly greased with coconut oil, press the mixture tightly and firmly into the pan. Cover lightly with plastic wrap and refrigerate for 2 hours. Gently cut into bars and store chilled in airtight container for up to 2 weeks.

POWERHOUSE BARS

With goji berries, hemp seeds, chia seed, and oats, these protein-packed bars are full of all kinds of nourishing ingredients that will keep you going strong all day long.

1 cup pecans

½ cup raw cashews

9 dates

¼ teaspoon salt

1 tablespoon coconut oil

½ cup certified gluten-free oats

½ cup goji berries

¼ cup hemp seeds

¼ cup chia seed

- Line an 8 × 8-inch baking pan with plastic wrap or lightly oil with coconut oil.

- Place the pecans, cashews, and five of the dates into a food processor and blend until evenly crumbly. Add the salt and the remaining dates and pulse until well combined and dates are evenly chopped. Transfer mixture into a large bowl and stir in the coconut oil to evenly coat. Fold in the oats, goji berries, hemp seeds, and chia seed. Press the mixture firmly into the prepared baking pan and refrigerate for 2 hours. Cut into bars and store in an airtight container in the refrigerator for up to 2 weeks.

CHERRY PIE BARS

YIELD: 8 SERVINGS

The taste is just like cherry pie but these little bars are actually pretty good for you! I recommend seeking out the highest-quality dried cherries (organic, unsulphured, with no added sugar) for these for the most authentic cherry-pie flavor.

2 cups raw cashews

1 cup dried cherries (not sweetened)

½ teaspoon salt

10 Medjool dates

- In a food processor, combine the cashews, cherries, and salt and blend until coarsely crumbled. Add in the dates and pulse until finely crumbled and the mixture easily comes together and stays together when squeezed.

- Shape the mixture into individual bars by shaping into a tight disk, or square, and then cutting gently with knife. Wrap individually in plastic wrap or foil. Alternatively, shape into balls for bite-size snacking. Store in airtight container in refrigerator for up to 2 weeks.

CHERRY CHOCOLATE ALMOND SNACK BARS

YIELD: 12 SERVINGS

Like a crunchy granola bar, these chocolate bars are a great pick-me-up when your energy is down. Be sure to use only kasha (toasted buckwheat) that is brown in color, rather than greenish. Kasha is usually located next to untoasted buckwheat groats, oftentimes in the bulk or natural foods sections.

1½ cups kasha (toasted buckwheat kernels), soaked for 2 hours

⅓ cup + 2 tablespoons cocoa powder

2 tablespoons chia seed

½ cup maple syrup

3 tablespoons date sugar

⅔ cup almond flour

½ teaspoon salt

½ cup dried cherries (not sweetened)

¼ teaspoon coconut or olive oil

* Preheat oven to 300°F. Line a baking tray with parchment paper.

- Drain the soaked kasha completely. In a large bowl, combine all of the ingredients except for the oil. Use the ¼ teaspoon coconut oil to grease clean hands and gently pat down the mixture into a rectangle, about ¼ to ½ inch thick. Bake for 30 minutes. Remove from oven, gently cut into squares using a spatula (but don't separate) and continue to bake for an additional 20 minutes. Let cool completely and then break into individual bars. Store in airtight container for up to 1 week.

If you can't locate toasted kasha, you can always toast your own at 300°F for 45 minutes, stirring often until browned.

FRUITY TREATS

PEANUT BUTTER BANANA ICE CREAM

YIELD: 2 CUPS

This recipe couldn't get any easier with only four ingredients, and it's good for you! Eat up.

5 very ripe bananas, peeled

½ cup smooth salted peanut butter

½ teaspoon vanilla extract

1 cup canned full-fat coconut milk

- Place all ingredients into a blender and blend until very smooth, for about 1 minute. Pour into the bowl of your ice cream maker and process according to manufacturer's instructions. Or, alternatively, freeze all ingredients in a bowl for 3 hours, and then immediately process in a food processor until smooth. Store in airtight container in freezer for up to 1 month.

FRESH FRUITSICLES

YIELD: ABOUT 5

These gorgeous pops will have you excited about eating fruit and keeping cool at the same time. I like the combo of the fruits listed below, but, along with the grapes, you could add in any chopped fruits you please. You'll need popsicle molds for these, or you can pour into silicone ice cube trays or even small paper cups.

1 cup grapes, red or green

1 kiwi, peeled and diced

⅓ cup chopped red raspberries

⅓ cup blueberries

- Place the grapes into a blender and puree until smooth. Transfer to a bowl and stir in the diced fruit. Pour the mixture into popsicle molds and add wooden sticks to the center. Freeze overnight and then enjoy. Store in freezer for up to 1 month.

FRUIT SALSA AND CINNAMON CRISPS

YIELD: 6 SERVINGS

A fun twist on an old favorite, serve these "chips and salsa" at your next gathering for a sweet—and healthy—surprise.

CINNAMON CHIPS

4 white corn tortillas

1 tablespoon olive oil

1 tablespoon agave

¼ teaspoon salt

¼ teaspoon cinnamon, or to taste

FRUIT SALSA

1 cup berries (raspberry + blackberry works great)

1 cup strawberries, greens left on

½ cup seedless grapes, any variety

Juice of 1 lime

1 apple, diced with seeds removed

1 kiwi, peeled and diced

- Preheat oven to 400°F. Stack the corn tortillas and cut into six even triangles. Spread the triangles in an even layer onto an ungreased cookie sheet, so that none of them are touching.

- In a small bowl, whisk together the olive oil, agave, and salt. Brush lightly onto each side of the tortilla triangle (this will get a little sticky) and sprinkle one side of the triangles with cinnamon. Bake for 7 minutes, flip, and bake for an additional 2 minutes. Let cool while you make the salsa.

- In a food processor, combine the berries, strawberries, grapes, and lime juice and pulse until the fruit has been chopped, but not pureed, for about five or six times. Combine with the diced apples and kiwi and serve with cinnamon crisps. Store in airtight container in refrigerator for up to 1 week.

PINEAPPLE "LAYER CAKES"

YIELD: 2 PERSONAL-SIZE CAKES

These little stacks are a fun twist on the conventional version of the dessert. Handle the pineapple rings with care, if using canned, or cut a little on the thick side if using fresh. Looking for some crunch? Try adding a thin layer of crushed walnuts or pecans on top of the cashew cream! You can locate vanilla bean paste in specialty shops such as Williams Sonoma, or simply sub in the same amount of vanilla extract.

8 pineapple rings

½ cup Sweet Cashew Cream

½ teaspoon vanilla bean paste

2 tablespoons Cherry Vanilla Compote

- Drain the pineapple rings by placing them in a single layer on a paper towel. Let rest for 10 minutes, or until the rings are relatively dry. In a small bowl, mix together the cashew cream with the vanilla bean paste.

- On the plate you wish to serve it, create an alternating stack of pineapple, cashew cream, pineapple, etc., finishing with a dollop of the Cherry Vanilla Compote.

APPLE NACHOS

YIELD: 4 SERVINGS

These are perfect for creating other variations!

3 crispy and slightly tart apples, such as Honeycrisp or Granny Smith

1 teaspoon lemon juice

3 tablespoons creamy peanut butter

¼ cup <u>Date Syrup</u>

¼ cup sliced almonds

¼ cup pecans, roughly chopped

¼ cup flaked or shredded unsweetened coconut

¼ cup cacao nibs

* Remove the core from each apple and slice them very thin (about ⅛-inch thickness), using a sharp knife. Arrange on a plate so that each apple has a good amount of surface exposed. Lightly spritz with the lemon juice.

* Melt the peanut butter in a small saucepan along with the date syrup until it is very runny and drizzle it onto the apple slices. Top the apples and peanut butter with the almonds and pecans, and then drizzle with the melted date syrup. Finally, top with unsweetened flaked coconut and cacao nibs. Enjoy these with your hands, just like real nachos. Serve immediately.

ALLERGY NOTE

To make nut-free, sub in toasted sunflower seeds for the almonds.

STRAWBERRY BANANA FRUIT LEATHER

YIELD: 6 SERVINGS

My kids go bananas for these wholesome snacks. I recommend using a dehydrator for best results, but you can also bake them in the oven at 200°F, spread out on a silicone mat, for several hours until dried.

2 medium very ripe (a few brown spots is desired) bananas

2 heaping cups fresh small strawberries, greens on

- Blend the fruit until smooth in a high-speed blender or food processor, scraping down sides as needed. The consistency should resemble a fruit smoothie. Spread out into a fruit leather mat fitted for your dehydrator. Spread thinly and evenly and then rap the tray on a flat surface a few times to remove any air bubbles.

- Set your dehydrator to 135°F and let it roll until the fruit is no longer tacky, for about 4 to 5 hours. If using a conventional oven, simply spread thinly onto a silicone mat and set oven to lowest temperature with the door slightly ajar. Bake for 3 to 4 hours, until no longer tacky.

- Gently peel up from the tray and place onto a cutting board. Using a pizza cutter, slice into large sections and then immediately roll up onto waxed paper, so that the fruit is completely covered. Enjoy immediately or store for up to 1 month in an airtight container.

SHAKES AND OTHER DRINKS

CARROT CAKE SMOOTHIE

YIELD: 2 SERVINGS

Indulge at breakfast time with this delish drink! It boasts the addition of blackstrap molasses, which is chock full of good stuff like copper, iron, calcium, and potassium.

1 large carrot, stems and top removed

1 large banana, peeled and frozen

3 dates

½ cup unsweetened almond milk

¾ cup cold water

½ teaspoon cinnamon

Dash nutmeg

Dash cloves

1 teaspoon blackstrap molasses

Place the first four ingredients in a blender and process until the banana is mostly blended. Add the water, spices, and molasses and blend until creamy. Thin to taste with additional cold water, if desired. Serve immediately.

PIÑA COLADA

This tastes so authentic you may expect to feel a bit tipsy while sipping; but, rest assured, this libation is quite good for you. It may even ward off colds with all that pineapple, which is very high in vitamin C!

1 large peeled frozen banana

⅛ cup coconut cream (from can of coconut milk)

4 pineapple rings (or about ½ cup canned pineapple)

¾ cup pineapple juice

1 teaspoon rum extract

* Blend all ingredients until very smooth in a high-speed blender. Serve immediately.

APPLE PIE MILKSHAKE

YIELD: 1 SERVING

Easier than apple pie, and good for you, too! This "milk shake" makes a perfectly indulgent breakfast or a late afternoon snack.

1½ bananas, chopped and frozen

⅔ cup apple cider (no sugar added)

⅓ cup pecans

½ teaspoon cinnamon

Dash nutmeg

- Combine all ingredients into a blender and mix until very smooth. Thin with a little extra apple cider or nondairy milk if desired.

- Serve immediately.

BLUEBERRY BLIZZARD MILKSHAKE

YIELD: 1 SERVING

Blueberries are full of antioxidants and lend a beautiful blue hue to this milk shake. And that's not the only healthy ingredient: it's sweetened with bananas.

½ cup fresh or frozen blueberries

1½ peeled and frozen bananas

1 teaspoon vanilla extract

1 cup non dairy milk (almond is best)

- Place all the ingredients into a blender and blend until completely smooth. Serve immediately with a thick straw.

METRIC CONVERSIONS

The recipes in this book have not been tested with metric measurements, so some variations might occur.

Remember that the weight of dry ingredients varies according to the volume or density factor: 1 cup of flour weighs far less than 1 cup of sugar, and 1 tablespoon doesn't necessarily hold 3 teaspoons.

General Formula for Metric Conversion

Ounces to grams   multiply ounces by 28.35

Grams to ounces   multiply ounces by 0.035

Pounds to grams   multiply pounds by 453.5

Pounds to kilograms   multiply pounds by 0.45

Cups to liters   multiply cups by 0.24

Fahrenheit to Celsius   subtract 32 from Fahrenheit

temperature, multiply by 5, divide by 9

Celsius to Fahrenheit   multiply Celsius temperature by 9,

divide by 5, add 32

Volume (Liquid) Measurements

1 teaspoon = ⅙ fluid ounce = 5 milliliters

1 tablespoon = ½ fluid ounce = 15 milliliters 2 tablespoons = 1 fluid ounce = 30 milliliters

¼ cup = 2 fluid ounces = 60 milliliters

⅓ cup = 2⅔ fluid ounces = 79 milliliters

½ cup = 4 fluid ounces = 118 milliliters

1 cup or ½ pint = 8 fluid ounces = 250 milliliters

2 cups or 1 pint = 16 fluid ounces = 500 milliliters

4 cups or 1 quart = 32 fluid ounces = 1,000 milliliters

1 gallon = 4 liters

Oven Temperature Equivalents, Fahrenheit (F) and Celsius (C)

100°F = 38°C

200°F = 95°C

250°F = 120°C

300°F = 150°C

350°F = 180°C

400°F = 205°C

450°F = 230°C

Volume (Dry) Measurements

¼ teaspoon = 1 milliliter

½ teaspoon = 2 milliliters

¾ teaspoon = 4 milliliters 1 teaspoon = 5 milliliters

1 tablespoon = 15 milliliters

¼ cup = 59 milliliters

⅓ cup = 79 milliliters

½ cup = 118 milliliters

⅔ cup = 158 milliliters

¾ cup = 177 milliliters 1 cup = 225 milliliters

4 cups or 1 quart = 1 liter

½ gallon = 2 liters 1 gallon = 4 liters

Linear Measurements

½ in = 1½ cm

1 inch = 2½ cm

6 inches = 15 cm

8 inches = 20 cm

10 inches = 25 cm

12 inches = 30 cm

20 inches = 50 cm